ADRENAL FATIGUE FACTS

50 QUESTIONS ABOUT ADRENAL FATIGUE ANSWERED!

(SIMPLIFIED)

By

Dr. Chris Allan

Table of Contents

INTRODUCTION

Do you feel tired all the time, even after a full night's rest? Are you struggling with mood swings, low libido, and weight gain? If so, you may be suffering from adrenal fatigue.

Adrenal fatigue is a condition that affects millions of people worldwide. It occurs when your adrenal glands, which produce hormones that regulate your body's response to stress, become overworked and can no longer keep up with the demands placed on them.

If you suspect that you may be suffering from adrenal fatigue, you probably have many questions about the condition, its causes, and how to treat it. That's where this book comes in.

Adrenal Fatigue Facts: 50 Questions Answered is the ultimate guide to understanding and managing adrenal fatigue. In this book, we answer the fifty most commonly asked questions about adrenal fatigue, providing you with the information you need to take control of your health and well-being.

So why are question and answers the fastest way to learn these facts? The answer is simple: questions force you to actively engage with the material, which makes it more likely that you will retain the information. When you read a question, your brain has to work to come up with an answer, which helps to reinforce the knowledge in your memory.

Additionally, the question and answer format of this book allows you to quickly and easily find the information you need. Instead of reading through dense paragraphs of text, you can simply flip to the question that interests you and read the answer. This makes it a perfect reference guide for busy people who don't have the time or patience to read through lengthy explanations.

But don't just take our word for it. Research has shown that question and answer formats are highly effective for learning and retention. In fact, a study published in the Journal of Educational Psychology found that students who studied using a question and answer format scored significantly higher on exams than those who studied using traditional methods.

So whether you're a healthcare professional looking to better understand adrenal fatigue or someone who is struggling with the condition, Adrenal Fatigue Facts: 50 Questions Answered is the book for you. With its clear and concise answers, you'll have all the information you need to take control of your health and start feeling your

best.

SECTION 1

KNOW ABOUT ADRENAL FATIGUE

1. What is adrenal fatigue, and how is it different from other medical conditions that affect the adrenal glands?

Adrenal fatigue is a term used to describe a collection of symptoms such as fatigue, weakness, and difficulty coping with stress. It is not a recognized medical condition, and there is no scientific evidence to support the notion that the adrenal glands become exhausted or fatigued from chronic stress.

There are several medical conditions that affect the adrenal glands, including adrenal insufficiency, Cushing's syndrome, and pheochromocytoma. Adrenal insufficiency occurs when the adrenal glands do not produce enough hormones, while Cushing's syndrome is caused by the overproduction of cortisol. Pheochromocytoma is a rare tumor that produces excess amounts of adrenaline and noradrenaline.

Unlike adrenal fatigue, these medical conditions are diagnosed through medical testing, such as blood and urine tests, imaging studies, and specialized hormone tests. Treatment for these conditions varies depending on the underlying cause and may include medications, surgery, or other interventions.

2. What are the adrenal glands, and what role do they play in the body?

The adrenal glands are small, triangular-shaped endocrine glands located above the kidneys. They consist of two main parts: the adrenal cortex and the adrenal medulla. Each of these parts plays a distinct role in regulating the body's physiological functions.

The adrenal cortex produces hormones that help regulate metabolism, immune system function, and the body's response to stress. The primary hormones produced by the adrenal cortex are corticosteroids, including cortisol, aldosterone, and androgens. Cortisol helps regulate the body's response to stress, by increasing blood sugar levels and suppressing the immune system. Aldosterone helps regulate blood pressure and electrolyte balance, by causing the kidneys to reabsorb sodium and excrete potassium. Androgens are male sex hormones, but they are also produced in females and play a role in the development of secondary sex characteristics.

The adrenal medulla produces two hormones: epinephrine (also known as adrenaline) and norepinephrine (also known as noradrenaline). These hormones are involved in the body's "fight or flight" response to stress, by increasing heart rate, dilating blood vessels, and stimulating the release of glucose from the liver.

Overall, the adrenal glands play a crucial role in regulating the body's response to stress, maintaining homeostasis, and supporting metabolism and immune function.

3. What causes adrenal fatigue, and are there any specific triggers that can make it worse?

While adrenal fatigue is not a recognized medical condition, the concept of adrenal dysfunction resulting from chronic stress is widely accepted. Chronic stress is the most common cause of adrenal fatigue. When the body is exposed to stress, the adrenal gland releases hormones, including cortisol and adrenaline, to help the body cope with the stressor. However, if stress is chronic, the adrenal gland may become overworked and eventually fail to produce enough hormones to meet the body's needs.

In addition to chronic stress, other factors that may contribute to adrenal fatigue include poor diet, lack of sleep, and chronic illness. Certain medications, such as corticosteroids, may also suppress adrenal function and contribute to adrenal fatigue.

There are several triggers that can make adrenal fatigue worse. These include ongoing stress, lack of sleep, poor diet, and physical overexertion. Other triggers may include exposure to environmental toxins, such as chemicals and heavy metals, and chronic infections.

It's important to note that the symptoms of adrenal fatigue are non-specific and can be caused by a variety of other medical conditions. Therefore, it's important to consult with a healthcare professional if you're experiencing symptoms of fatigue, anxiety, or sleep disturbances. A healthcare professional can help determine the underlying cause of your symptoms and develop an appropriate treatment plan.

4. How common is adrenal fatigue, and who is most likely to develop this condition?

Many people report symptoms that they associate with adrenal fatigue, such as fatigue, difficulty concentrating, and disrupted sleep patterns.

It is difficult to estimate how common adrenal fatigue is because there is no universally accepted diagnostic criteria for the condition. Some estimates suggest that it may affect as many as 80% of people at some point in their lives, but these numbers are difficult to verify.

There is no clear consensus on who is most likely to develop adrenal fatigue, but some factors may increase the risk of experiencing symptoms associated with the condition. These factors may include chronic stress, a history of trauma or abuse, poor diet and nutrition, lack of exercise, and certain medical conditions or medications.

It is worth noting that many of the symptoms associated with adrenal fatigue are also commonly associated with other medical conditions, such as depression, anxiety, thyroid disorders, and sleep apnea. Therefore, it is important to seek medical advice if you are experiencing persistent or severe symptoms, rather than self-diagnosing based on the concept of adrenal fatigue.

5. Can stress be a significant factor in the development of adrenal fatigue, and if so, how?

Stress can certainly play a significant role in the development of adrenal fatigue. When we experience stress, our bodies release hormones, including cortisol, from the adrenal glands. Cortisol is important for regulating blood sugar, blood pressure, and inflammation, and helps us respond to stress.

However, when we experience chronic stress, the adrenal glands can become overworked and may struggle to produce adequate levels of cortisol. This can lead to a condition commonly referred to as adrenal fatigue.

Additionally, chronic stress can also lead to other issues that can contribute to adrenal fatigue. For example, chronic stress can disrupt our sleep patterns, which can further impact cortisol levels and the health of our adrenal glands. Chronic stress can also lead to inflammation, which can damage the adrenal glands and impair their function.

It is important to note that the concept of adrenal fatigue is not widely recognized in the medical community, and some experts believe that the term is misleading and inaccurate. However, the impact of chronic stress on the body, including the adrenal glands, is well-established. Therefore, it is important to take steps to manage stress and support overall health in order to prevent the negative effects of chronic stress on the body.

6. What are the symptoms of adrenal fatigue, and how do they differ from those of other conditions?

Some individuals who report experiencing symptoms associated with "adrenal fatigue" may describe feeling constantly tired or exhausted, even after getting enough rest. They may also experience difficulty falling asleep or staying asleep, as well as a general lack of energy or motivation to engage in everyday activities.

Other symptoms may include frequent illnesses, such as colds or flu, as well as digestive issues such as bloating, constipation, or diarrhea. Some individuals may also report experiencing anxiety or depression, difficulty concentrating, or mood swings.

It is important to note that these symptoms may also be associated with other conditions, such as thyroid disorders, chronic fatigue syndrome, or depression. Therefore, it is essential to seek medical advice to determine the underlying cause of these symptoms and to receive appropriate treatment.

Overall, if you are experiencing any of these symptoms, it is important to prioritize self-care, such as getting enough rest, eating a balanced diet, and engaging in regular exercise, and to consult with a healthcare professional to determine the underlying cause of your symptoms and to receive appropriate treatment.

7. What are some of the tests that doctors use to diagnose adrenal fatigue, and how accurate are these tests?

There are several tests that may be used to diagnose adrenal fatigue. These include:

Salivary cortisol test: This test measures the level of cortisol, a hormone produced by the adrenal glands, in the saliva. Proponents of adrenal fatigue theory suggest that levels of cortisol may be abnormally low in people with adrenal fatigue.

ACTH stimulation test: This test measures how the adrenal glands respond to a hormone called adrenocorticotropic hormone (ACTH), which is produced by the pituitary gland. The test involves giving an injection of ACTH and then measuring the levels of cortisol in the blood.

DHEA-S test: This test measures the level of dehydroepiandrosterone sulfate (DHEA-S), another hormone produced by the adrenal glands. Some practitioners suggest that low levels of DHEA-S may be a sign of adrenal fatigue.

However, there is limited scientific evidence to support the accuracy of these tests for diagnosing adrenal fatigue. In fact, some experts argue that the tests may be misleading or inconclusive. Moreover, many of the symptoms associated with adrenal fatigue, such as fatigue, weight gain, and muscle weakness, are also common in many other conditions.

8. Can a poor diet contribute to the development of adrenal fatigue, and if so, which types of foods should be avoided?

Yes, a poor diet can contribute to the development of adrenal fatigue. Adrenal fatigue is often associated with chronic stress and overuse of the adrenal glands, which can lead to a depletion of cortisol and other hormones. Poor dietary choices can exacerbate this condition by placing additional stress on the body and impairing the ability of the adrenal glands to function optimally.

To support healthy adrenal function, it is important to consume a well-balanced diet that includes plenty of fresh fruits and vegetables, lean proteins, and healthy fats. On the other hand, there are some types of foods that should be avoided or limited to promote adrenal health. These include:

Processed foods: Processed foods are often high in sugar, unhealthy fats, and sodium, which can contribute to inflammation, weight gain, and other health issues that place additional stress on the body.

Caffeine: Caffeine is a stimulant that can increase cortisol levels, which can further tax the adrenal glands and exacerbate symptoms of adrenal fatigue.

Alcohol: Alcohol can disrupt the body's natural sleep patterns, leading to poor quality sleep and further impairing adrenal function.

High-glycemic foods: Foods that are high in sugar or refined carbohydrates can cause blood sugar spikes and crashes, which can lead to fatigue and stress on the body.

Artificial sweeteners: Artificial sweeteners can disrupt the body's natural hormone balance and increase inflammation, which can further impair adrenal function.

By making healthy dietary choices and avoiding or limiting these types of foods, individuals can support healthy adrenal function and reduce the risk of developing adrenal fatigue. It is important to consult with a healthcare provider to determine the best approach to managing this condition.

9. How does sleep affect adrenal function, and what can be done to improve sleep quality in people with adrenal fatigue?

Sleep plays a critical role in regulating adrenal function. The adrenal glands are responsible for producing hormones such as cortisol, which help regulate the body's stress response. When we are sleep-deprived, cortisol levels can become dysregulated, leading to a variety of health problems.

Lack of sleep can lead to an overactive adrenal response, which can cause chronic fatigue, anxiety, and difficulty managing stress. Additionally, chronic sleep deprivation can also suppress the immune system, leading to an increased risk of illness and disease.

To improve sleep quality in people with adrenal issues, it's important to establish healthy sleep habits. This includes setting a regular sleep schedule, avoiding caffeine and alcohol before bed, creating a comfortable sleep environment, and practicing relaxation techniques such as meditation or deep breathing.

In addition to improving sleep quality, it's also important to address any underlying issues that may be contributing to adrenal dysfunction. This may involve working with a healthcare professional to address nutritional deficiencies, manage stress levels, and develop a personalized treatment plan.

Overall, prioritizing healthy sleep habits and addressing underlying issues can help improve adrenal function and overall health.

10. Are there any natural remedies or supplements that can help support adrenal health and reduce the symptoms of adrenal fatigue?

There are natural remedies and supplements that can support adrenal health and help reduce the symptoms that may be associated with it.

Adaptogenic herbs: These herbs are thought to help the body adapt to stress and support healthy adrenal function.

Some examples include ashwagandha, rhodiola, and holy basil.

Vitamin C: This antioxidant vitamin is involved in the production of adrenal hormones, and supplementation may help support adrenal health.

B-complex vitamins: These vitamins are important for energy production and stress management, and a deficiency can contribute to adrenal dysfunction.

Magnesium: This mineral is involved in over 300 enzymatic reactions in the body, including those related to energy production and stress management.

Sleep: Getting adequate sleep is crucial for adrenal health, as sleep deprivation can lead to increased cortisol levels and adrenal dysfunction.

Stress reduction techniques: Engaging in activities such as yoga, meditation, and deep breathing can help reduce stress and support healthy adrenal function.

It is important to note that while these natural remedies and supplements may help support adrenal health and reduce symptoms, they should not be used as a replacement for medical treatment. If you are experiencing symptoms that may be related to adrenal dysfunction, it is important to consult with a healthcare provider for proper diagnosis and treatment.

11. Can exercise help improve adrenal function, or does it exacerbate symptoms in people with adrenal fatigue?

Exercise can have both positive and negative effects on adrenal function, depending on the individual and the specific circumstances. In general, exercise is known to be beneficial for overall health, including the functioning of the adrenal glands. Regular exercise can help to reduce stress levels, which is important because the adrenal glands play a key role in regulating the body's response to stress.

However, it's important to note that people with certain conditions, such as adrenal insufficiency or Addison's disease, may need to take extra precautions when exercising. These conditions involve a malfunctioning or damaged adrenal gland, which can affect the body's ability to produce important hormones like cortisol. In such cases, strenuous exercise may exacerbate symptoms and put additional stress on the adrenal glands, potentially causing further damage.

In general, it's recommended that people with any health condition, including those affecting the adrenal glands, consult with a healthcare provider before starting a new exercise routine. This can help ensure that any potential risks are identified and addressed, and that the exercise program is tailored to the individual's specific needs and abilities.

In summary, regular exercise can be beneficial for overall adrenal function and stress management. However, individuals with certain adrenal-related conditions may need to take extra precautions when exercising, and should consult with a healthcare provider before starting a new exercise routine.

12. How long does it typically take to recover from adrenal fatigue, and are there any specific steps that should be taken during this recovery process?

There is no definitive answer to how long it takes to recover from adrenal fatigue, as the condition can vary widely in severity and the underlying causes can be complex. However, the recovery process usually involves a combination of lifestyle changes, dietary modifications, and targeted supplements or medications.

Some specific steps that can help support adrenal function and promote recovery include:

Reducing stress: Chronic stress is a major contributor to adrenal fatigue, so finding ways to reduce stress is key. This might involve practicing relaxation techniques such as meditation or yoga, getting regular exercise, or prioritizing sleep.

Eating a balanced diet: A diet that is rich in whole foods, including plenty of fruits and vegetables, lean protein, and healthy fats, can help support adrenal function and reduce inflammation.

Supplementing with key nutrients: Certain nutrients, such as vitamin C, B vitamins, magnesium, and adaptogenic herbs like ashwagandha or rhodiola, may help support adrenal function and reduce fatigue.

Working with a healthcare professional: It's important to work with a healthcare professional who can help identify and address any underlying health conditions that may be contributing to adrenal fatigue, as well as provide guidance on lifestyle modifications and supplements.

Therefore, recovery from adrenal fatigue can be a gradual process, and may require patience and perseverance. By making targeted lifestyle and dietary changes and working with a knowledgeable healthcare provider, however, many people are able to successfully recover and regain their energy and vitality.

13. Can medication help treat adrenal fatigue, or is a holistic approach more effective?

Some alternative medicine practitioners use the term adrenal fatigue to describe a collection of symptoms they attribute to the adrenal glands not functioning properly.

If one is experiencing the symptoms of adrenal fatigue, the most effective approach is to consult a healthcare professional. Some practitioners may recommend medication, such as corticosteroids or thyroid hormone replacement therapy, to manage the symptoms of adrenal insufficiency. However, the appropriate treatment will depend on the underlying cause of the symptoms, which may require further diagnostic testing.

It is important to note that a holistic approach can also be beneficial for managing symptoms associated with adrenal fatigue. This may include stress management techniques, such as meditation and yoga, dietary changes, and lifestyle modifications, such as getting enough sleep and exercise. These approaches may help to reduce stress levels and promote overall well-being.

Ultimately, the effectiveness of any treatment approach will depend on the individual and their unique circumstances. It is important to work with a qualified healthcare provider to determine the most appropriate course of action for managing symptoms associated with adrenal fatigue, and to carefully consider the risks and benefits of any proposed treatments.

14. What are some of the long-term consequences of untreated adrenal fatigue, and how can these be prevented?

One of the most significant consequences of untreated adrenal dysfunction is chronic fatigue, which can severely impact a person's quality of life. Other potential consequences include disrupted sleep patterns, cognitive impairment, mood disorders, and weakened immune function. Over time, these issues can lead to chronic diseases such as cardiovascular disease, diabetes, and autoimmune disorders.

To prevent these long-term consequences, it's essential to identify and address any underlying health issues that may be contributing to adrenal dysfunction. This may include managing stress levels, improving sleep habits, adopting a healthy diet and exercise routine, and treating any underlying medical conditions such as thyroid disorders or chronic infections. In some cases, supplements or medications may be prescribed to support adrenal function and manage symptoms.

It's also essential to work with a qualified healthcare provider who can help you identify the root cause of your symptoms and develop an individualized treatment plan. With proper care and attention, it's possible to prevent the long-term consequences of adrenal dysfunction and restore your overall health and well-being.

15. Can adrenal fatigue be prevented, or is it an inevitable consequence of modern living?

While it may be difficult to completely prevent all factors that can contribute to fatigue and stress, there are steps that can be taken to minimize their impact. For example, practicing stress-reducing activities like meditation or yoga, eating a balanced and nutritious diet, getting regular exercise, and prioritizing adequate sleep are all important for maintaining overall health and well-being. Additionally, it's important to pay attention to your body and listen to its signals. If you are feeling consistently fatigued or experiencing other symptoms that are impacting your daily life, it may be a sign that you need to make changes to your lifestyle or seek medical advice.

Overall, while there may not be a surefire way to completely prevent all factors that can contribute to fatigue and stress, taking proactive steps to manage stress, prioritize self-care, and listen to your body can go a long way in maintaining your health and well-being.

16. How does the hormonal balance in the body contribute to adrenal fatigue, and can hormone therapy help treat this condition?

One theory is that chronic stress can lead to dysregulation of the body's hormonal system, including the hypothalamic-pituitary-adrenal (HPA) axis, which plays a key role in regulating the body's response to stress.

The adrenal glands, which sit on top of the kidneys, produce a variety of hormones, including cortisol, adrenaline, and noradrenaline, which are involved in the body's stress response. When the body is under stress, the HPA axis is activated, leading to the release of cortisol, which helps to mobilize energy and cope with the stressor.

However, prolonged exposure to stress can lead to dysregulation of the HPA axis and a state of chronically elevated cortisol levels. This can contribute to adrenal fatigue, which is characterized by symptoms such as fatigue, difficulty sleeping, anxiety, and digestive problems.

Hormone therapy is sometimes used to treat adrenal fatigue, but its effectiveness is controversial and not well-supported by scientific evidence. Some practitioners may prescribe cortisol or other hormones to help regulate the HPA axis and reduce symptoms of adrenal fatigue. However, there is concern that hormone therapy can disrupt the body's natural hormone balance and lead to other health problems.

In general, the best approach to managing adrenal fatigue is to address the underlying causes of stress and promote healthy lifestyle habits such as exercise, healthy eating, and stress management techniques. In some cases, supplements such as adaptogenic herbs or vitamins may be helpful in supporting the body's natural stress response. However, it's important to work with a qualified healthcare provider to develop an individualized treatment plan that takes into account your unique symptoms and health history.

17. Is there a link between adrenal fatigue and mental health conditions, such as anxiety or depression?

Chronic stress can lead to dysregulation of the hypothalamic-pituitary-adrenal (HPA) axis, which plays a role in the body's stress response. This dysregulation can cause changes in cortisol levels, which may contribute to the development of anxiety or depression.

It's important to note that anxiety and depression are complex conditions that can have many causes, including genetic, environmental, and psychological factors. Chronic stress and dysregulation of the HPA axis can contribute to the development of these conditions, but they are unlikely to be the sole cause.

It's also worth noting that some medical conditions, such as thyroid disorders or hormonal imbalances, can cause symptoms that overlap with those attributed to adrenal fatigue. Therefore, it's important to consult a medical professional for an accurate diagnosis and appropriate treatment plan.

In summary, while there may be a link between chronic stress and dysregulation of the HPA axis with anxiety and depression, the concept of adrenal fatigue is not widely accepted in mainstream medicine, and more research is needed to fully understand the relationship between stress and mental health.

18. Can acupuncture or other alternative therapies help treat adrenal fatigue, and if so, how?

Acupuncture is a traditional Chinese medicine technique that involves inserting fine needles into specific points on the body. According to Chinese medicine, acupuncture can help balance the flow of qi, or life energy, through the body, which can help alleviate a variety of symptoms, including fatigue.

Some practitioners of alternative medicine believe that acupuncture can help regulate the hypothalamic-pituitary-adrenal (HPA) axis, which plays a role in regulating the body's stress response. According to this theory, acupuncture can help reduce stress and improve the function of the adrenal glands, which could help alleviate the symptoms associated with adrenal fatigue.

Other alternative therapies that some people believe can help with adrenal fatigue include herbal supplements, dietary changes, and stress reduction techniques like meditation and yoga. However, there is little scientific evidence to support the effectiveness of these therapies for treating adrenal fatigue.

Definitely, the efficacy of alternative therapies for treating adrenal fatigue is a subject of debate and controversy in the medical community. It is important to discuss any treatment options with a qualified healthcare provider before attempting to use them.

19. Are there any foods or drinks that can help support adrenal function and reduce the risk of developing adrenal fatigue?

The adrenal glands are responsible for producing hormones that help regulate various bodily functions, including stress response, metabolism, and blood pressure. While there is no specific diet or magic food that can prevent or cure adrenal fatigue, some foods and drinks can support adrenal function and overall health.

High-quality protein: Protein is essential for building and repairing tissues, and it also helps regulate hormone production. Eating high-quality sources of protein such as grass-fed beef, wild-caught fish, organic chicken, and eggs can help support adrenal function.

Healthy fats: Healthy fats are necessary for the production of hormones, and they also help reduce inflammation. Sources of healthy fats include avocados, coconut oil, olive oil, nuts, and seeds.

Complex carbohydrates: Complex carbohydrates provide energy and help regulate blood sugar levels. Examples of complex carbohydrates include whole grains, fruits, and vegetables.

Vitamin C-rich foods: Vitamin C is essential for adrenal function, and it also has antioxidant properties. Foods high in vitamin C include citrus fruits, strawberries, kiwi, bell peppers, broccoli, and kale.

Herbal teas: Certain herbal teas such as licorice root, ashwagandha, and ginseng have been shown to support adrenal function and reduce stress.

Magnesium-rich foods: Magnesium is essential for energy production, and it also helps regulate blood sugar levels and reduce stress. Foods high in magnesium include leafy greens, nuts, seeds, and whole grains.

It's important to note that while certain foods and drinks can support adrenal function and overall health, they cannot cure or prevent adrenal fatigue. Adrenal fatigue is a controversial and unproven condition, and the best way to support adrenal health is to maintain a healthy lifestyle with a balanced diet, regular exercise, and stress management techniques.

20. What role do lifestyle factors, such as smoking or alcohol consumption, play in the development of adrenal fatigue?

There is some evidence to suggest that lifestyle factors such as smoking or alcohol consumption may play a role in the development of adrenal fatigue. Adrenal fatigue is a controversial and poorly defined condition that is not recognized as a medical diagnosis by most mainstream medical organizations. However, it is often used as a catch-all term to describe a variety of non-specific symptoms such as fatigue, difficulty concentrating, and sleep disturbances.

Some studies have suggested that smoking may contribute to adrenal fatigue by increasing oxidative stress and inflammation in the body, which can lead to damage to the adrenal glands. Smoking has also been linked to a higher risk of developing autoimmune disorders, which can affect the functioning of the adrenal glands. Similarly, alcohol consumption has been shown to increase oxidative stress and inflammation in the body, and may also contribute to the development of autoimmune disorders.

Other lifestyle factors that may contribute to adrenal fatigue include poor diet, lack of exercise, chronic stress, and inadequate sleep. These factors can all lead to chronic activation of the stress response system, which can eventually lead to dysfunction of the adrenal glands.

It is important to note that the concept of adrenal fatigue is not widely accepted by the medical community, and there is limited scientific evidence to support its existence as a distinct condition. Therefore, it is unclear to what extent lifestyle factors may contribute to its development. However, it is well established that lifestyle factors such as smoking and alcohol consumption can have negative effects on overall health and well-being, and should be avoided or minimized where possible.

21. How can people with adrenal fatigue manage their symptoms and maintain their quality of life?

Individuals who experience symptoms such as fatigue, difficulty sleeping, and stress may benefit from strategies to manage these symptoms and maintain their quality of life. Here are some tips that may be helpful:

Prioritize sleep: Aim to get 7-8 hours of restful sleep each night. Develop a bedtime routine that promotes relaxation, such as taking a warm bath, reading a book, or meditating.

Manage stress: Incorporate stress-management techniques such as meditation, deep breathing exercises, or yoga into your daily routine. Avoid over-exertion, and take breaks throughout the day to rest and recharge.

Eat a balanced diet: Eat a nutrient-dense diet that includes plenty of fruits, vegetables, whole grains, and lean proteins. Limit caffeine, sugar, and processed foods, which can contribute to fatigue and disrupt sleep.

Stay hydrated: Drink plenty of water and limit alcohol and caffeine, which can dehydrate the body.

Exercise regularly: Engage in regular physical activity, such as walking, cycling, or swimming. Exercise can help reduce stress, improve mood, and boost energy levels.

Consider supplementation: Some individuals may benefit from supplements such as magnesium, vitamin D, and probiotics. However, it is important to speak with a healthcare professional before starting any new supplement regimen.

Seek support: Connect with friends, family, or a therapist to help manage stress and cope with any emotional challenges related to your symptoms.

While these strategies may help manage symptoms and improve quality of life, it is important to consult a healthcare professional for a proper diagnosis and treatment plan.

22. Are there any support groups or online communities that can provide advice and encouragement for people with adrenal fatigue?

Yes, there are many support groups and online communities that can provide advice and encouragement for people with adrenal fatigue. These groups can be helpful in sharing experiences, providing emotional support, and offering practical advice on managing symptoms.

Some examples of online support communities for adrenal fatigue include Facebook groups such as "Adrenal Fatigue & Related Disorders Support Group" and "Adrenal Fatigue Support Group," as well as forums such as "Adrenal Fatigue Forum" and "Adrenal Fatigue Solution Community." These groups are typically moderated by individuals with personal experience of adrenal fatigue and/or medical professionals with knowledge of the condition.

In addition to online support communities, there are also many resources available for those seeking information and advice on adrenal fatigue. These include websites such as the "Adrenal Fatigue Solution" and "Adrenal Fatigue Society," which offer information on symptoms, diagnosis, and treatment options for adrenal fatigue.

It's important to note that while online support groups and resources can be helpful in managing adrenal fatigue, it's always advisable to seek medical advice from a qualified healthcare professional. Adrenal fatigue can be a complex condition, and an accurate diagnosis and tailored treatment plan can be key to managing symptoms effectively.

23. How do healthcare providers treat adrenal fatigue, and are there any controversies surrounding this condition within the medical community?

Some healthcare providers consider adrenal fatigue to be a legitimate condition caused by chronic stress, while others do not recognize it as a legitimate diagnosis.

For healthcare providers who do recognize adrenal fatigue as a condition, treatment typically involves lifestyle changes and supplements. The goal of treatment is to reduce stress and support the adrenal glands, which are believed to be overworked in people with adrenal fatigue.

Some lifestyle changes that may be recommended include stress-reduction techniques like meditation or yoga, dietary changes, exercise, and adequate sleep. Supplements that may be recommended include adaptogenic herbs like ashwagandha, vitamins and minerals like vitamin B and magnesium, and probiotics.

It's important to note that there is limited scientific evidence to support the effectiveness of these treatments for adrenal fatigue. Some healthcare providers may recommend hormone replacement therapy, such as cortisol or DHEA, but this approach is controversial and not widely accepted.

In general, the controversy surrounding adrenal fatigue arises from a lack of clear diagnostic criteria and limited scientific evidence to support the concept. Some healthcare providers argue that the symptoms associated with adrenal fatigue may be caused by other underlying medical conditions or lifestyle factors, and that treating adrenal fatigue may not be effective in these cases.

24. Can adrenal fatigue be cured completely, or is it a chronic condition that requires ongoing management?

It is important to note that the treatment and prognosis of any medical condition depend on the underlying cause and severity of the condition. In some cases, lifestyle changes such as stress reduction, diet modification, and exercise may be sufficient to alleviate symptoms and prevent recurrence.

However, in more severe cases, medical treatment may be necessary. For example, if adrenal insufficiency is the underlying cause of symptoms, hormone replacement therapy may be needed to restore adrenal function. In some cases, other underlying medical conditions may need to be addressed before symptoms of adrenal fatigue can be resolved.

It is important to note that chronic stress can have a negative impact on overall health and well-being, and stress reduction strategies may be important for long-term management of any related symptoms. This may include techniques such as meditation, yoga, or therapy.

In conclusion, if adrenal fatigue is a real medical condition, the prognosis and treatment options will depend on the underlying cause and severity of symptoms. In some cases, it may be possible to completely resolve symptoms, while in others, ongoing management may be necessary. It is always important to consult with a qualified medical professional to determine the best course of treatment for any medical condition.

25. What can be done to raise awareness of adrenal fatigue and help people understand this condition better?

Raising awareness of adrenal fatigue can be done in several ways:

Education: People can be educated about adrenal fatigue through various means such as online resources, books, seminars, webinars, workshops, and public lectures. This education should focus on the causes, symptoms, and treatments of the condition.

Social media campaigns: Social media platforms such as Twitter, Facebook, and Instagram can be utilized to raise awareness of adrenal fatigue. Creating hashtags, sharing informative posts, and organizing online chats are some ways to spread awareness.

Community outreach: Organizing community events such as health fairs, workshops, and conferences can help to educate the public about adrenal fatigue. This can be done in collaboration with healthcare providers, patient advocacy groups, and other stakeholders.

Collaboration with healthcare providers: Healthcare providers can play a crucial role in raising awareness of adrenal fatigue. They can educate their patients about the condition and its treatments, as well as provide resources for further education and support.

Media coverage: Media coverage can help to raise awareness of adrenal fatigue on a larger scale. This can be done through articles, TV shows, podcasts, and other media outlets.

In summary, raising awareness of adrenal fatigue can be achieved through education, social media campaigns, community outreach, collaboration with healthcare providers, and media coverage. By increasing understanding of this condition, we can help people receive the proper diagnosis, treatment, and support they need.

SECTION 2

TREATMENT OPTIONS

26. What are some conventional treatment options for adrenal fatigue?

Adrenal fatigue, also known as adrenal insufficiency, is a condition in which the adrenal glands are not producing enough hormones, particularly cortisol. Conventional treatment options for adrenal fatigue include:

Lifestyle changes: Lifestyle changes such as reducing stress, improving sleep, and engaging in regular exercise can help improve the function of the adrenal glands.

Dietary changes: A healthy diet can also support adrenal function. Eating a balanced diet that includes lean protein, whole grains, and fruits and vegetables can help to stabilize blood sugar levels, which can in turn support the adrenal glands.

Supplements: Certain supplements such as B vitamins, magnesium, and adaptogenic herbs like ashwagandha and rhodiola can help support adrenal function.

Hormone replacement therapy: In cases where adrenal insufficiency is severe, hormone replacement therapy may be necessary. This involves taking synthetic cortisol or other hormones to replace those that the adrenal glands are not producing.

Medications: In rare cases, medications such as hydrocortisone or fludrocortisone may be prescribed to help support adrenal function.

It is important to note that the concept of adrenal fatigue is controversial within the medical community, and some experts do not recognize it as a medical condition. Some of the symptoms attributed to adrenal fatigue, such as fatigue and low energy, can have other underlying causes and should be evaluated by a healthcare professional. In addition, any treatment for adrenal fatigue should be supervised by a healthcare professional to ensure that it is safe and effective.

27. Are there any medications that can help manage adrenal fatigue symptoms?

If someone is experiencing symptoms that they attribute to adrenal fatigue, there may be some medications that can help manage those symptoms. However, the medications prescribed will depend on the specific symptoms being experienced, as well as any underlying medical conditions that may be contributing to those symptoms.

For example, if someone is experiencing fatigue, a doctor may prescribe a stimulant medication, such as modafinil or methylphenidate, to help increase energy levels. If someone is experiencing anxiety or depression, a doctor may prescribe an antidepressant or anti-anxiety medication, such as selective serotonin reuptake inhibitors (SSRIs) or benzodiazepines.

However, it is important to note that these medications do not treat the underlying cause of the symptoms, and they may have potential side effects or risks. It is also important to work closely with a doctor to determine the best course of treatment for individual needs, and to avoid self-diagnosis and self-treatment.

In conclusion, while there is no scientific evidence to support the concept of adrenal fatigue as a distinct medical condition, there may be medications that can help manage the symptoms associated with it. However, the specific medications prescribed will depend on the individual symptoms and underlying medical conditions, and it is important to work closely with a doctor to determine the best course of treatment.

28. Can lifestyle changes such as diet and exercise improve adrenal fatigue?

Adrenal fatigue is a term used to describe a group of nonspecific symptoms that are believed to be caused by chronic stress and a disruption of the normal functioning of the adrenal glands. While not officially recognized as a medical diagnosis, many people seek to alleviate symptoms associated with adrenal fatigue through lifestyle changes such as diet and exercise.

Diet plays a crucial role in the management of adrenal fatigue. A diet rich in nutrient-dense whole foods, including plenty of fruits, vegetables, and lean proteins, can help support the body's natural stress response and energy levels. Adequate hydration and avoiding processed foods, caffeine, and alcohol can also help reduce stress on the adrenal glands. Additionally, supplementing with adaptogenic herbs, such as ashwagandha and rhodiola, may help support the body's stress response.

Exercise is also an essential component of managing adrenal fatigue. Engaging in regular physical activity can help reduce stress and improve mood. However, it's important to be mindful of not overexerting oneself, as intense exercise can be stressful on the body and worsen symptoms of adrenal fatigue. Incorporating gentle exercises, such as yoga or walking, into a daily routine may be more beneficial.

In addition to diet and exercise, stress management techniques, such as mindfulness meditation, deep breathing exercises, and adequate sleep, can also be helpful in managing symptoms of adrenal fatigue. Addressing underlying emotional stressors and seeking support from a healthcare provider or therapist may also be necessary for long-term management of adrenal fatigue.

It's important to note that while lifestyle changes may be helpful in managing symptoms associated with adrenal fatigue, the term "adrenal fatigue" is not widely accepted in the medical community. If experiencing persistent symptoms, it's essential to consult with a healthcare provider to rule out any underlying medical conditions and receive appropriate treatment.

29. What role does stress management play in treating adrenal fatigue?

Adrenal fatigue is a term used to describe a collection of symptoms that some people believe occur when the adrenal glands are unable to keep up with the demands of stress. While the concept of adrenal fatigue is controversial in the medical community, stress management can play an important role in treating the symptoms that people attribute to this condition.

When the body experiences stress, the adrenal glands release hormones like cortisol and adrenaline to help the body cope. Over time, chronic stress can lead to an overworked adrenal system, which can cause fatigue, difficulty sleeping, and other symptoms.

Stress management techniques like meditation, deep breathing, and yoga can help to reduce the impact of stress on the body, and in turn, reduce the demands placed on the adrenal glands. Additionally, getting enough rest, eating a healthy diet, and exercising regularly can also help to support adrenal function.

It is important to note that while stress management can help to alleviate the symptoms of adrenal fatigue, it is not a substitute for medical treatment. If you are experiencing symptoms that you believe may be related to adrenal fatigue, it is important to speak with a healthcare professional who can provide a proper diagnosis and treatment plan.

30. Can hormone replacement therapy (HRT) be used to treat adrenal fatigue?

Adrenal fatigue is not an accepted medical diagnosis, and its existence as a medical condition is still a topic of debate. Therefore, there are no established treatment protocols or medications for adrenal fatigue. Hormone replacement therapy (HRT) is used to treat specific medical conditions such as menopause, hypogonadism, and some cancers.

HRT replaces hormones that the body may no longer produce in sufficient quantities. The use of HRT may be helpful in treating the symptoms associated with low levels of certain hormones. However, the use of HRT in adrenal fatigue is not supported by scientific evidence, and it may not be appropriate or effective.

The adrenal glands produce several hormones, including cortisol, adrenaline, and aldosterone. These hormones play important roles in regulating various body functions, such as blood pressure, metabolism, and stress response. In some medical conditions, such as Addison's disease, the adrenal glands do not produce enough cortisol and require medical treatment. However, in cases where adrenal function is not impaired, there is no evidence to support the use of HRT.

In conclusion, there is no evidence to suggest that HRT is an effective treatment for adrenal fatigue. If you have concerns about your adrenal function or are experiencing symptoms, it is recommended to speak to a healthcare provider to rule out any underlying medical conditions.

31. What are some herbal remedies that are commonly used to treat adrenal fatigue?

Some herbal remedies are believed to be helpful in relieving its symptoms.

Licorice root: Licorice root contains compounds that mimic the effects of cortisol, a hormone produced by the adrenal glands, and can help to support adrenal function. It is often taken in the form of a tea or supplement.

Ashwagandha: Ashwagandha is an adaptogenic herb that is believed to help the body cope with stress and reduce fatigue. It can be taken in the form of a supplement or added to food or drinks as a powder.

Rhodiola rosea: Rhodiola rosea is another adaptogenic herb that has been used to support adrenal function and reduce stress. It can be taken in supplement form or added to food or drinks as a powder.

Panax ginseng: Panax ginseng is an adaptogenic herb that is believed to help improve energy levels, reduce stress, and support adrenal function. It can be taken in supplement form or added to food or drinks as a powder.

Holy basil: Holy basil is an adaptogenic herb that has been used to reduce stress and improve energy levels. It can be taken in supplement form or added to food or drinks as a powder.

It is important to note that while herbal remedies may be helpful in relieving the symptoms of adrenal fatigue, they should not be used as a substitute for medical treatment.

If you are experiencing persistent fatigue or other symptoms, it is important to consult with a healthcare professional to rule out any underlying medical conditions.

32. How effective is licorice root in treating adrenal fatigue?

Licorice root has been traditionally used in Ayurvedic and Chinese medicine for its medicinal properties. It is considered effective in treating adrenal fatigue due to its active component, glycyrrhizin, which has been shown to increase the cortisol levels in the body. Cortisol is a hormone produced by the adrenal glands that helps the body to respond to stress.

When the body experiences stress, the adrenal glands release cortisol to help the body cope with stress. In adrenal fatigue, the adrenal glands are unable to produce enough cortisol, leading to fatigue, weakness, and other symptoms. Licorice root helps to increase cortisol levels, which can alleviate the symptoms of adrenal fatigue.

Licorice root also contains flavonoids and saponins, which have anti-inflammatory properties. Inflammation is a common symptom of adrenal fatigue, and reducing inflammation can help to alleviate symptoms such as fatigue and brain fog.

Additionally, licorice root has been shown to have a beneficial effect on the digestive system. It can soothe the digestive tract, reduce inflammation, and promote the growth of beneficial bacteria in the gut. Adrenal fatigue can lead to digestive issues, and licorice root can help to alleviate these symptoms.

However, it's important to note that licorice root should be taken under the guidance of a healthcare professional. High doses of licorice root can lead to side effects such as high blood pressure and low potassium levels. Pregnant women and people with certain medical conditions, such as liver disease, should avoid licorice root.

In summary, licorice root can be effective in treating adrenal fatigue due to its ability to increase cortisol levels, reduce inflammation, and promote digestive health. However, it should be taken under the guidance of a healthcare professional to ensure safe and effective use.

33. How does ashwagandha help with adrenal fatigue?

Ashwagandha, also known as Withania somnifera, is a traditional Ayurvedic herb that has been used for centuries in Indian medicine to treat various health issues. One of its most well-known benefits is its ability to help alleviate symptoms of adrenal fatigue.

Adrenal fatigue is a condition in which the adrenal glands, located above the kidneys, are unable to produce sufficient amounts of cortisol, a hormone that helps the body cope with stress. This can lead to symptoms such as fatigue, insomnia, anxiety, and depression.

Ashwagandha has been shown to help improve adrenal function by reducing cortisol levels in the body. It contains compounds called adaptogens, which help the body adapt to stress by regulating the production of cortisol. By doing so, it can help reduce symptoms of adrenal fatigue and promote overall wellbeing.

Studies have found that ashwagandha supplementation can lead to significant reductions in cortisol levels, as well as improvements in sleep quality, anxiety, and overall stress levels. It has also been shown to help boost energy levels and improve overall physical performance.

In addition to its effects on cortisol levels, ashwagandha also has antioxidant and anti-inflammatory properties, which can help protect against cellular damage and reduce inflammation throughout the body. This can help support overall immune function and promote optimal health.

Overall, ashwagandha is a powerful herb that can help alleviate symptoms of adrenal fatigue and promote overall health and wellbeing. However, as with any supplement, it's important to consult with a healthcare professional before starting to take ashwagandha to ensure it's safe for you and won't interact with any medications you may be taking.

34. What is the recommended dosage of maca for treating adrenal fatigue?

Maca is a root vegetable that is native to Peru and is widely used as a supplement for various health benefits, including improving energy levels and reducing stress. Adrenal fatigue is a controversial condition that is not recognized by many medical professionals. However, some people believe that maca can be useful in treating the symptoms of adrenal fatigue, which include fatigue, brain fog, and difficulty coping with stress.

There is no standard recommended dosage of maca for treating adrenal fatigue because the condition is not well-defined, and the research on maca's effectiveness for this purpose is limited. However, some experts suggest taking maca in doses of 1.5-5 grams per day, preferably in the morning or early afternoon. It is recommended to start with a low dose and gradually increase it to assess tolerance.

Maca is available in various forms, including capsules, powders, and extracts. It is important to choose a high-quality maca supplement from a reputable source to ensure that it is pure and potent. Maca may interact with certain medications and may not be suitable for people with thyroid disorders. Therefore, it is advisable to consult a healthcare professional before taking maca or any other supplement, especially if you have any underlying medical conditions.

It is worthy of note that, while maca may have some potential benefits for treating the symptoms of adrenal fatigue, more research is needed to confirm its effectiveness. Additionally, it is important to approach any supplement with caution and to consult a healthcare professional before taking it, especially if you have any underlying health conditions or are taking any medications.

35. Can ginseng be used to treat adrenal fatigue?

Ginseng has been traditionally used in Chinese medicine for its various health benefits, including improving energy levels and reducing stress. While there is no scientific evidence to support the concept of adrenal fatigue as a medical diagnosis, some people claim that ginseng can help alleviate the symptoms associated with this condition.

Adrenal fatigue is a term used to describe a collection of nonspecific symptoms such as fatigue, body aches, and nervousness that are believed to be caused by chronic stress and the subsequent depletion of the adrenal glands. However, there is no medical consensus on whether adrenal fatigue is a real condition, and it is not recognized as a medical diagnosis.

While ginseng has been shown to have various benefits, including improving cognitive function, reducing inflammation, and increasing energy levels, there is little scientific evidence to support the use of ginseng specifically for adrenal fatigue. Some studies have suggested that ginseng may help reduce stress levels and improve physical endurance, which could potentially help alleviate some of the symptoms associated with adrenal fatigue. However, more research is needed to determine the effectiveness of ginseng for this purpose.

It is important to note that ginseng is not a substitute for medical treatment, and anyone experiencing persistent or severe symptoms should consult a healthcare provider. In addition, ginseng can interact with certain medications and may not be safe for everyone, especially pregnant or breastfeeding women, children, and individuals with certain medical conditions such as diabetes, high blood pressure, or autoimmune disorders.

36. Is rhodiola rosea effective in treating adrenal fatigue?

Rhodiola Rosea is a herb that is commonly used in traditional medicine to manage a variety of conditions, including stress and fatigue. It is believed to work by regulating the body's stress response, reducing inflammation, and enhancing cognitive function. There is some evidence to suggest that rhodiola rosea may be effective in treating symptoms related to adrenal fatigue, but more research is needed to confirm its effectiveness.

Adrenal fatigue is a condition characterized by chronic fatigue, difficulty sleeping, and a range of other symptoms that are thought to be caused by an imbalance in the body's adrenal hormones. While adrenal fatigue is not a recognized medical condition, it is believed to be a consequence of chronic stress and can lead to significant impairments in daily life.

Rhodiola rosea has been shown to improve physical and mental performance in healthy individuals and may also help to reduce fatigue and improve mood in people with stress-related conditions. Some studies have suggested that rhodiola rosea can improve adrenal function and reduce the symptoms of adrenal fatigue. However, the evidence is limited and more research is needed to determine its effectiveness for this purpose.

As a matter of fact, while rhodiola rosea may have potential in treating some symptoms related to adrenal fatigue, it should not be considered a replacement for medical treatment or advice. If you are experiencing symptoms of fatigue or stress, it is important to consult with a healthcare professional to determine the underlying cause and appropriate treatment.

37. What is the recommended dosage of holy basil for adrenal fatigue?

Holy basil, also known as Tulsi, is an herb commonly used in Ayurvedic medicine for its adaptogenic and anti-inflammatory properties. It has been traditionally used to help alleviate stress and improve overall wellness, which can be beneficial in the context of adrenal fatigue.

There is no specific recommended dosage of holy basil for adrenal fatigue as it is not a medically recognized condition. Adrenal fatigue is a term used by alternative medicine practitioners to describe a collection of nonspecific symptoms, such as fatigue, difficulty sleeping, and difficulty handling stress, which they believe to be caused by chronic stress and an overtaxed adrenal gland. However, the scientific community does not recognize adrenal fatigue as a legitimate medical diagnosis.

That being said, holy basil is generally considered safe for most people when taken in moderation. It is available in various forms, including capsules, teas, and extracts. The appropriate dosage may vary depending on the specific product and individual factors such as age, health status, and other medications being taken.

If you are interested in taking holy basil, it is recommended that you speak with a healthcare professional before doing so. They can help you determine a safe and appropriate dosage based on your individual needs and health status. Additionally, it is important to remember that holy basil should not be used as a substitute for medical treatment for any specific medical condition, including adrenal fatigue, without the guidance of a healthcare professional.

38. Are there any fruits or vegetables that can help alleviate adrenal fatigue symptoms?

Certain dietary changes may help alleviate symptoms associated with chronic stress.

Fruits and vegetables are an essential part of a healthy diet, providing vitamins, minerals, and antioxidants that can help support the body's immune system and reduce inflammation. Some fruits and vegetables may be particularly helpful in reducing symptoms associated with chronic stress.

Leafy green vegetables such as spinach, kale, and collard greens are rich in magnesium, a mineral that plays a vital role in regulating the body's stress response. Magnesium can help reduce anxiety and promote relaxation by regulating the production of cortisol, the primary stress hormone produced by the adrenal glands.

Berries such as blueberries, strawberries, and raspberries are rich in antioxidants, which can help reduce inflammation in the body. Chronic stress can lead to chronic inflammation, which can contribute to a range of health problems, including depression, anxiety, and autoimmune disorders.

Citrus fruits such as oranges, grapefruits, and lemons are rich in vitamin C, a nutrient that can help reduce the production of cortisol and other stress hormones. Vitamin C is also essential for the proper functioning of the adrenal glands.

Other fruits and vegetables that may be helpful in reducing symptoms associated with chronic stress include avocados, bananas, sweet potatoes, and cruciferous vegetables such as broccoli and cauliflower. These foods are rich in nutrients that can help support the body's immune system and reduce inflammation, which can contribute to overall health and well-being.

39. How does omega-3 fatty acids help with adrenal fatigue?

Omega-3 fatty acids are a type of polyunsaturated fat that are important for overall health and well-being. They are found in high concentrations in fatty fish such as salmon, mackerel, and sardines, as well as in some nuts and seeds.

One of the ways in which omega-3 fatty acids can help with adrenal fatigue is by reducing inflammation in the body. Inflammation is a natural response to injury or infection, but chronic inflammation can contribute to a variety of health problems, including adrenal fatigue. Omega-3s have anti-inflammatory properties that can help to reduce inflammation and promote healing.

Another way in which omega-3s can help with adrenal fatigue is by supporting the health of the adrenal glands themselves. The adrenal glands are responsible for producing hormones that help to regulate the body's response to stress. When the body is under stress for extended periods of time, the adrenal glands can become fatigued and less able to produce these hormones.

Omega-3s can help to support the health of the adrenal glands and improve their function.

Omega-3s may also be helpful for reducing symptoms of anxiety and depression, which are commonly associated with adrenal fatigue. Studies have shown that omega-3 supplementation can improve mood and reduce symptoms of anxiety and depression in some people.

It's important to note that while omega-3s can be helpful for supporting overall health and well-being, they are not a cure for adrenal fatigue. If you are experiencing symptoms of adrenal fatigue, it's important to consult with a healthcare provider for a proper diagnosis and treatment plan.

40. Can magnesium supplements help with adrenal fatigue?

Adrenal fatigue is a term used to describe a collection of symptoms that occur when the adrenal glands function below normal levels. Symptoms may include fatigue, weakness, difficulty concentrating, and difficulty handling stress. Magnesium is an essential mineral that plays a vital role in many bodily functions, including energy metabolism and the regulation of the stress response.

Although magnesium supplementation may be beneficial for some people with adrenal fatigue, the evidence is limited and inconclusive. Some studies suggest that magnesium supplementation may improve energy levels and reduce stress in individuals with mild to moderate adrenal fatigue, but other studies have not found significant benefits.

Magnesium helps to regulate the stress response by reducing the release of stress hormones like cortisol and adrenaline. It also plays a role in energy production by supporting the metabolism of glucose, the body's primary source of fuel. Magnesium is also involved in the production of ATP, the molecule that provides energy for cellular processes.

Magnesium supplementation may be helpful for individuals with adrenal fatigue who have low levels of magnesium. However, it is important to note that high doses of magnesium can cause adverse effects such as diarrhea, nausea, and stomach cramps. Therefore, it is recommended to consult a healthcare provider before starting magnesium supplementation, especially if you have any underlying medical conditions or are taking medications.

In conclusion, magnesium supplementation may provide some benefits for individuals with adrenal fatigue, but the evidence is limited and inconclusive. It is important to address the underlying causes of adrenal fatigue, such as stress management and lifestyle changes, in addition to considering magnesium supplementation. Consulting a healthcare provider before starting any new supplement or treatment is always recommended.

41. Is vitamin C beneficial for treating adrenal fatigue?

Vitamin C is an essential nutrient that plays a crucial role in many physiological processes, including the immune response, collagen synthesis, and antioxidant defense. Some studies suggest that vitamin C supplementation may help reduce the negative effects of stress on the body, including the dysregulation of the HPA axis and the subsequent disruption of adrenal hormone production. In one study, participants who took vitamin C supplements for two weeks showed a significant reduction in cortisol levels, a hormone that is commonly elevated in individuals with chronic stress.

While these findings are promising, it is important to note that vitamin C supplementation alone is unlikely to be a cure-all for adrenal fatigue or chronic stress. Adopting a healthy lifestyle that includes regular exercise, a balanced diet, stress management techniques, and adequate sleep is key to supporting overall adrenal function and reducing the negative effects of chronic stress on the body.

In summary, while the evidence supporting the use of vitamin C for treating adrenal fatigue is limited, there is some evidence to suggest that it may be beneficial in reducing the negative effects of chronic stress on the body. However, it is important to adopt a holistic approach to managing adrenal fatigue and prioritize lifestyle factors that support overall health and well-being.

42. What role does vitamin D play in adrenal fatigue?

Vitamin D is an essential nutrient that plays several crucial roles in the body, including promoting bone health, supporting the immune system, and regulating mood. Additionally, research has suggested that vitamin D may also play a role in adrenal fatigue.

Adrenal fatigue is a condition characterized by a collection of symptoms that may include fatigue, sleep disturbances, difficulty coping with stress, and decreased immune function. While not recognized as a medical condition by all healthcare professionals, some believe that adrenal fatigue may result from prolonged stress or chronic illness, which can cause the adrenal glands to function sub-optimally.

One of the ways that vitamin D may impact adrenal fatigue is through its effects on the immune system. Research has shown that vitamin D helps regulate immune function by promoting the production of antimicrobial peptides that help fight infections. In addition, vitamin D has been shown to help regulate inflammation in the body, which may be beneficial in reducing symptoms associated with adrenal fatigue.

Another way that vitamin D may impact adrenal fatigue is through its effects on mood. Low levels of vitamin D have been linked to an increased risk of depression and other mood disorders. Since adrenal fatigue can also cause mood disturbances, maintaining adequate levels of vitamin D may be important in supporting overall mood and well-being.

Furthermore, vitamin D plays a role in the regulation of cortisol, a hormone produced by the adrenal glands that is involved in the body's response to stress. Some studies have suggested that vitamin D supplementation may help regulate cortisol levels, which may be beneficial in managing symptoms of adrenal fatigue.

In summary, while the exact role of vitamin D in adrenal fatigue is still being studied, research has suggested that maintaining adequate levels of this nutrient may be important in supporting immune function, regulating mood, and managing stress levels. However, it is always important to consult with a healthcare professional before making any changes to your supplement regimen.

43. Is B-complex vitamin supplementation recommended for adrenal fatigue?

B-complex vitamins are a group of essential water-soluble vitamins that play a crucial role in energy metabolism and nervous system function. They are also important in the production of hormones and neurotransmitters, which may be affected in individuals with adrenal fatigue.

While some alternative health practitioners may recommend B-complex vitamin supplementation for individuals with adrenal fatigue, there is limited scientific evidence to support this practice.

In fact, excessive intake of B-complex vitamins can lead to adverse effects, such as nausea, vomiting, and diarrhea. Additionally, some individuals may have underlying medical conditions that require medical attention, and self-diagnosing and treating with supplements can delay appropriate treatment.

If you are experiencing fatigue or other non-specific symptoms, it is recommended to consult with a healthcare professional for an accurate diagnosis and appropriate treatment. They can also provide guidance on nutritional supplementation, if necessary, based on your individual needs and medical history.

In summary, while B-complex vitamins are essential for overall health, there is limited scientific evidence to support their use for adrenal fatigue. If you are experiencing symptoms, it is recommended to seek medical attention and guidance on appropriate treatment options.

44. How does iron deficiency affect adrenal fatigue?

Iron is an essential mineral that plays a critical role in the production of red blood cells, which carry oxygen throughout the body. Adrenal fatigue, on the other hand, is a term used to describe a collection of symptoms that occur when the adrenal glands function below the optimal level. The adrenal glands produce a variety of hormones, including cortisol, which helps the body to respond to stress.

Iron deficiency can have a negative impact on adrenal function, as the adrenal glands require iron to produce hormones. Specifically, iron is necessary for the production of cortisol, which is important for managing stress. When the body is under stress, cortisol levels rise to help the body cope with the demands being placed upon it. However, in the absence of sufficient iron, the adrenal glands may not be able to produce enough cortisol, which can lead to adrenal fatigue.

Iron deficiency can also lead to anemia, which is a condition in which there are not enough red blood cells to carry oxygen throughout the body. Anemia can cause fatigue, weakness, and other symptoms that are similar to those associated with adrenal fatigue. Furthermore, iron deficiency can impair immune function, making it more difficult for the body to fight off infections and other health challenges.

To prevent iron deficiency and its potential impact on adrenal function, it is important to consume a diet that is rich in iron. Foods such as red meat, poultry, fish, beans, and leafy green vegetables are all good sources of iron. Iron supplements may also be recommended in some cases, particularly for individuals who are at risk of developing iron deficiency. If you suspect that you may be experiencing adrenal fatigue or iron deficiency, it is important to speak with your healthcare provider to receive an accurate diagnosis and appropriate treatment.

45. Are there any natural supplements that can improve adrenal gland function?

The adrenal glands are responsible for producing hormones that help the body respond to stress, regulate blood pressure, and maintain blood sugar levels. When the adrenal glands are not functioning optimally, individuals may experience symptoms such as fatigue, weakness, and a weakened immune system. While there are no specific natural supplements that can improve adrenal gland function, there are several that may be beneficial for supporting overall adrenal health.

Ashwagandha: Ashwagandha is an adaptogenic herb that has been used for centuries in Ayurvedic medicine to help the body cope with stress. Research suggests that it may help reduce cortisol levels, the hormone released in response to stress, and improve overall adrenal gland function.

Rhodiola: Rhodiola is another adaptogenic herb that has been used to help the body adapt to stress. It may help improve adrenal gland function by reducing cortisol levels and improving the body's response to stress.

Licorice root: Licorice root contains compounds that may help support adrenal function by increasing the production of cortisol. However, it is important to note that long-term use of licorice root may lead to high blood pressure and other health issues, so it should be used with caution.

Vitamin C: Vitamin C is an important nutrient for adrenal health, as it helps the body produce cortisol and other hormones. It also acts as an antioxidant, protecting the adrenal glands from oxidative stress.

B-complex vitamins: B vitamins are essential for energy production and adrenal function. Vitamin B5, in particular, is important for adrenal health, as it is involved in the production of adrenal hormones.

It is important to note that while these natural supplements may be beneficial for supporting adrenal health, they should not be used as a replacement for medical treatment. If you are experiencing symptoms of adrenal dysfunction, it is important to consult with a healthcare professional to determine the underlying cause and develop an appropriate treatment plan.

46. What is the recommended dosage of adaptogenic herbs for adrenal fatigue?

Adaptogenic herbs are a class of herbs that help the body adapt to stress and support overall well-being. They are believed to be particularly helpful for individuals experiencing adrenal fatigue, a condition where the adrenal glands become exhausted from chronic stress.

The recommended dosage of adaptogenic herbs for adrenal fatigue may vary depending on the specific herb, individual needs, and severity of the condition. It is important to consult with a qualified healthcare provider or a licensed herbalist before starting any new supplement regimen.

Some commonly used adaptogenic herbs for adrenal fatigue include Ashwagandha, Rhodiola, Ginseng, Holy Basil, and Licorice root.

Ashwagandha, for example, is often taken in doses of 300-500mg per day, while Rhodiola is typically taken in doses of 200-600mg per day. Ginseng is often taken in doses of 100-400mg per day, while Holy Basil is typically taken in doses of 500-1000mg per day. Licorice root can be taken as a tea or in capsule form, and the recommended dose can vary depending on the product.

It is important to note that adaptogenic herbs may take time to build up in the body and show their full effects, and it is generally recommended to take them for at least several weeks to see results. It is also important to monitor for any potential side effects or interactions with other medications or supplements.

In addition to taking adaptogenic herbs, individuals experiencing adrenal fatigue may benefit from lifestyle changes such as reducing stress, getting enough sleep, and engaging in regular exercise. A balanced and nutritious diet can also help support adrenal health.

47. Can acupuncture help alleviate adrenal fatigue symptoms?

Adrenal fatigue is a condition characterized by chronic fatigue, low energy, brain fog, and a disrupted sleep pattern, among other symptoms. Acupuncture is an alternative therapy that has been used to treat various ailments, including chronic fatigue, anxiety, and depression, which are also symptoms of adrenal fatigue. Acupuncture involves the insertion of thin needles into specific points on the body to stimulate the flow of energy, or Qi. According to traditional Chinese medicine, adrenal fatigue is caused by a deficiency or imbalance of Qi. Acupuncture aims to rebalance the body's energy, which in turn can alleviate symptoms of adrenal fatigue.

Acupuncture may help alleviate adrenal fatigue symptoms by reducing stress levels. Stress is a significant contributor to adrenal fatigue, and acupuncture has been shown to reduce stress hormones, such as cortisol, in the body. Acupuncture may also stimulate the production of endorphins, which are natural painkillers that can help improve mood and reduce fatigue.

Acupuncture can also improve sleep quality, which is essential for individuals with adrenal fatigue. Studies have shown that acupuncture can increase the production of melatonin, a hormone that regulates the sleep-wake cycle.

In conclusion, acupuncture may help alleviate symptoms of adrenal fatigue by reducing stress levels, improving sleep quality, and rebalancing the body's energy. However, more research is needed to determine the effectiveness of acupuncture as a treatment for adrenal fatigue, and it should not be used as a substitute for conventional medical treatment. It is always recommended to consult with a healthcare provider before starting any new treatment.

48. What are some relaxation techniques that can help manage adrenal fatigue?

Adrenal fatigue is a condition that occurs when the adrenal glands are overworked, leading to a variety of symptoms such as fatigue, sleep disturbances, brain fog, and difficulty concentrating. It is often caused by chronic stress, which can lead to a decrease in the production of cortisol, the hormone responsible for regulating stress in the body. There are several relaxation techniques that can help manage adrenal fatigue, including:

Deep breathing: Deep breathing techniques involve taking slow, deep breaths from the diaphragm. This helps to activate the parasympathetic nervous system, which helps to reduce stress and promote relaxation.

Progressive muscle relaxation: Progressive muscle relaxation involves tensing and then releasing each muscle group in the body, starting from the toes and working up to the head. This helps to release tension in the muscles and promote relaxation.

Meditation: Meditation involves focusing on the breath or a specific word or phrase to quiet the mind and promote relaxation. It has been shown to reduce stress and improve overall well-being.

Yoga: Yoga combines physical postures, breathing techniques, and meditation to promote relaxation and reduce stress. It has been shown to improve adrenal function and reduce cortisol levels.

Massage therapy: Massage therapy involves the manipulation of the soft tissues in the body to promote relaxation and reduce stress. It has been shown to reduce cortisol levels and improve overall well-being.

Aromatherapy: Aromatherapy involves the use of essential oils to promote relaxation and reduce stress. Essential oils such as lavender, chamomile, and bergamot have been shown to be particularly effective.

In summary, there are several relaxation techniques that can help manage adrenal fatigue. These include deep breathing, progressive muscle relaxation, meditation, yoga, massage therapy, and aromatherapy. By incorporating these techniques into your daily routine, you can help to reduce stress and promote relaxation, which can help to improve adrenal function and reduce symptoms of adrenal fatigue.

49. Can massage therapy be beneficial for adrenal fatigue?

Adrenal fatigue is a condition where the adrenal glands are unable to produce sufficient amounts of hormones such as cortisol, which are essential for managing stress. Symptoms of adrenal fatigue include fatigue, difficulty sleeping, weight gain, and irritability. While there is no conclusive evidence that massage therapy can cure adrenal fatigue, there are indications that it may be beneficial in managing symptoms.

Massage therapy can help reduce stress levels, which is a significant contributing factor to adrenal fatigue. When we experience stress, our body produces cortisol, which is responsible for the "fight or flight" response. Prolonged stress can cause the adrenal glands to become overworked, leading to adrenal fatigue. Massage therapy can help reduce stress by relaxing the body and mind, which can help regulate cortisol levels and prevent overstimulation of the adrenal glands.

Massage therapy can also improve circulation, which can help nourish the adrenal glands and reduce inflammation. The adrenal glands require a steady supply of oxygen and nutrients to function correctly. Massage therapy can help increase blood flow to the adrenal glands, which can help nourish them and reduce inflammation. This, in turn, can help reduce the strain on the adrenal glands, allowing them to produce hormones more efficiently.

In conclusion, while massage therapy is not a cure for adrenal fatigue, it can be beneficial in managing symptoms by reducing stress levels and improving circulation. It is essential to consult with a healthcare professional to develop a comprehensive treatment plan that includes massage therapy along with other therapies, such as dietary changes, exercise, and stress management techniques, to manage adrenal fatigue effectively.

50. What is the recommended duration of treatment for adrenal fatigue with natural remedies?

Adrenal fatigue is a condition characterized by chronic fatigue, body aches, and low blood pressure, which is believed to be caused by prolonged stress. While there is no definitive diagnosis or treatment for adrenal fatigue recognized by mainstream medicine, some natural remedies have been recommended to alleviate the symptoms of this condition.

It's important to note that there is no consensus among natural health practitioners about the recommended duration of treatment for adrenal fatigue. Some suggest that treatment should last for several months, while others recommend long-term lifestyle changes that are sustained over a period of years.

The natural remedies that are often recommended for adrenal fatigue include:

Dietary changes: It is essential to eat a nutrient-dense diet that is rich in whole foods, especially vegetables and fruits. Avoiding caffeine, sugar, and processed foods can also help to reduce stress on the adrenal glands.

Herbal supplements: Adaptogenic herbs such as Ashwagandha, Rhodiola, and Licorice root can help to improve adrenal function and reduce stress.

Lifestyle changes: Incorporating stress-reducing practices such as meditation, yoga, and deep breathing into your daily routine can help to support the adrenal glands.

Rest and relaxation: Getting enough sleep is essential for the body to heal and restore itself. It is recommended to aim for 7-8 hours of sleep per night and to practice relaxation techniques before bed.

It's important to note that natural remedies may take time to work, and it's essential to be patient and consistent with the recommended treatment plan. It's also important to work with a qualified healthcare professional who can monitor your progress and provide guidance on the duration of treatment that is best for your individual

needs.

Here are 30 facts about Adrenal Fatigue you need to know.

1. Adrenal fatigue is not recognized as a medical diagnosis by most mainstream medical organizations.

2. It is a condition that is controversial and not universally accepted by medical professionals.

3. Adrenal fatigue is also known as hypothalamic-pituitary-adrenal (HPA) axis dysfunction.

4. The adrenal glands are located on top of the kidneys and are responsible for producing hormones that regulate many bodily functions.

5. Adrenal fatigue is characterized by a group of non-specific symptoms, such as fatigue, brain fog, difficulty sleeping, and body aches.

6. It is believed to be caused by chronic stress, which over time can cause the adrenal glands to become

overworked and eventually unable to produce adequate amounts of hormones.

7. Some alternative healthcare practitioners believe that adrenal fatigue is a real condition that can be diagnosed and treated.

8. Mainstream medicine suggests that the symptoms associated with adrenal fatigue are due to other medical conditions or lifestyle factors, such as depression, anxiety, or poor sleep habits.

9. The symptoms of adrenal fatigue are often similar to those of other medical conditions, making it difficult to diagnose.

10. There are no laboratory tests that can diagnose adrenal fatigue, and the diagnosis is usually based on a patient's symptoms and medical history.

11. Adrenal fatigue is not recognized by the American Medical Association or the American Association of Clinical Endocrinologists.

12. The concept of adrenal fatigue is often associated with alternative healthcare and is not well known among conventional medical practitioners.

13. Some practitioners of alternative healthcare suggest that adrenal fatigue can be treated with dietary changes, supplements, and lifestyle modifications.

14. There is little scientific evidence to support the idea that adrenal fatigue is a real condition.

15. Some experts believe that adrenal fatigue is a form of burnout, in which chronic stress leads to physical and emotional exhaustion.

16. Adrenal fatigue is often associated with chronic fatigue syndrome and fibromyalgia.

17. The symptoms of adrenal fatigue can be difficult to distinguish from those of other conditions, such as depression or hypothyroidism.

18. Many people who believe they have adrenal fatigue may actually have other medical conditions that require treatment.

19. Adrenal fatigue is not a condition that can be diagnosed with a single test or exam.

20. The symptoms associated with adrenal fatigue are not specific to the condition and can be caused by a variety of factors.

21. Some practitioners of alternative healthcare suggest that adrenal fatigue can be treated with herbs, such as ashwagandha and licorice root.

22. The use of herbs to treat adrenal fatigue is not supported by scientific evidence.

23. Some practitioners of alternative healthcare suggest that adrenal fatigue can be treated with supplements, such as vitamins B and C, magnesium, and zinc.

24. The use of supplements to treat adrenal fatigue is not supported by scientific evidence.

25. The symptoms of adrenal fatigue can vary widely from person to person.

26. Some people with adrenal fatigue may experience only mild symptoms, while others may be severely affected.

27. Adrenal fatigue is often associated with chronic stress and is more common in people who have high-stress jobs or lifestyles.

28. Adrenal fatigue is not considered to be a serious medical condition, but it can be disruptive to a person's life.

29. The symptoms associated with adrenal fatigue can be managed with lifestyle changes, such as reducing stress and getting enough sleep.

30. Some people with adrenal fatigue may benefit from psychotherapy or other forms of counseling to help them cope with stress.

Dr. Chri Allan wishes you Good Health!

....

Good Job on the completion of this book!

Knowledge is Power!

Now that you are aware, you are out of the trap of fear!

You may want to read any of my other books

HEALTHY HABITS FOR MEN!

HEALTHY HABITS FOR WOMEN!

NOTIFICATION FATIGUE!

PSORIASIS FACTS

KNOW THE FACS ABOUT CANCER

Check them out!